Weight Loss Surgery Success

Dr. V's A-Z Steps for Losing Weight and Gaining Enlightenment

Dr. Duc C. Vuong

FOR MY FATHER, WHOSE SPIRIT STILL
GUIDES ME EVERYDAY

INTRODUCTION

This is not your typical weight loss surgery book. It does not discuss the usual topics such as the types of weight loss surgery, insurance coverage, complications, or cooking recipes. There are many other books which touch on those subjects, and I even wrote some of them myself. This book complements those other books by considering *what really matters*. It deals less with your changing body and more with your changing mind, because to be successful after weight loss surgery you must expand your mind by stepping out of your comfort zone. You must discard the same old information and learn something new because *weight loss surgery success is primarily a mind game.*

I suggest you read this book all at once, then go back and read one letter each day. For that day, reflect on the message and try to incorporate its lesson into your life. This will give you approximately one month's worth of lessons. Then repeat the process, and turn it into habit. Carry this book with you wherever you go for a quick read whenever you have a free moment—when you are in line, when sitting at a restaurant table, or when commuting on the subway. Although it's compact and concise, the lessons have deeper meanings than you may at first realize; so dwell on them awhile. Let the messages linger some in your mind by reflecting on them throughout the day. Try reading them out loud, especially in front of a mirror. This is a powerful technique for manifesting all the things you really desire in your life.

Before you begin, let me set the scene by telling you my story:

In 2011, I began a personal journey to find Enlightenment, although I didn't realize it was Enlightenment I was searching for at the time. All roads since then have led me to the writing of this book. After Hurricane Ike tore through my community in 2008, I could not get my surgical practice back on track. So in 2011, I closed down my private practice in Houston and took a job at a wonderful hospital in a little town in southern Illinois with a population of only 6700 people. This position gave me the stability to regain my emotional and psychological footing as I spent many days and nights reading spiritual books, watching videos, and contemplating my place in this world. I read texts on spirituality, leadership, physics, Buddhism, and Taoism. I began to meditate. I learned to change the way I viewed past and present events in my life, and slowly over time my inner turmoil began to ease. I became more peaceful inside. I found happiness and contentment. I finally started sleeping through the night and waking up energetic. I learned many previously hidden life principles, and the more I practiced these principles, the more blessings came into my life. Now I am sharing some of these principles with you in this book.

Best wishes,

Dr. V

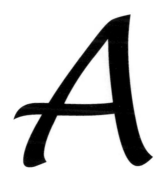

ATTITUDE

"Attitude is a little thing that makes a big difference."

– Winston Churchill

A stands for **Attitude**. Your attitude will determine how you see the world, whether you see your glass as half-empty or half-full. Focus on having only a positive attitude towards your weight loss surgery. Realize that everything in your life needed to happen in order for you to have the life you have today, even the events that might have contributed to your obesity. Rather than viewing your life as "jinxed" or "cursed," consider past events as lessons that had to be learned at the University of Life or at the "school of hard knocks".

Your attitude will also affect your aspirations. If your attitude is poor, then your aspirations will likely be small, when the truth is there are no limits to your aspirations. Most people have aspirations, but their aspirations are usually so small and uninspiring. Stop setting "realistic goals." Instead, why not see how high you can fly? Like the renowned motivational speaker Les Brown said, "Shoot for the stars, so if you fail, you might hit the moon!" Stop staring into the bottom of that half-empty glass, and start drinking from the half-full glass of life.

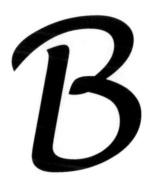

BE BETTER

"He who knows best knows how little he knows."

– Thomas Jefferson

B is for **Be Better**. Don't try to "do your best" every time. That does not leave room for improvement, and it lulls you into a false sense of security. "I did my best, so what more could I possibly do?" gives you comfort that if you didn't achieve your goal, it's okay because at least you tried your best. But there is really no way to know whether or not we actually did our "best." Rather than simply trying your best, decide to *be better*. Be better this time than last; be better today than you were yesterday. If yesterday was five diet sodas, you can be better today by drinking only four diet sodas, and then three tomorrow. You don't need to go straight from five to zero in a day, as long as every day you're getting better and better. You will be making progress in the right direction and will ultimately reach your weight loss goals if you simply resolve to be better today than yesterday.

But understand that Be Better also applies to every area of your life, not just weight loss. Be a better mother, spouse, or daughter. Be a better employee, coworker, or friend. Be a better gardener, cook, or runner this year than last year. To be better, you must learn new skills. The tricks that worked 10 years ago, no longer work today. Do not react to situations in the same way you did when you were 16. You must grow. You must evolve. Do not stay the same. Do not become complacent. The great philosopher Carl Jung said, "Our problems cannot be solved. They must be outgrown." This means you have to be better.

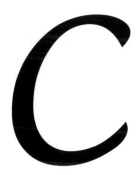

COMPASSION AND CHANGE

"If you want others to be happy, practice compassion.
If you want to be happy, practice compassion."

– Dalai Lama

C stands for **Compassion**. Without compassion, you will likely live a small and incomplete life. This is because you will be too wrapped up in your own weight loss troubles to see the true wonder of the world and the important role you play in it. Without compassion, you cannot be at peace with the new thinner and healthier you, because the world that we experience is just a reflection of our inner selves. Do you experience the world as kind or hostile? Loving or cruel? Compassionate or critical? Practicing compassion is easy— it can be as simple as giving a homeless beggar a word of kindness rather than a critical judgment. Perform one act of compassion towards another person today.

C also stands for Change. You can't change *out there* without changing *in here*; or as Jim Rohn said, "If you want your life to change, then *you* must change." Some patients wrongly think that after weight loss surgery they will be the exact same person just in a smaller body. But make no mistake: as you lose weight, things *will* change, you will change. Everything *must* change. If you don't change, then it won't be long before the old you returns. Change one thing about yourself today—be it a new haircut, an item of clothing, or a word you use to describe yourself.

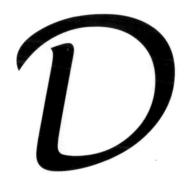

DREAM BIG DREAMS

"Dream no small dreams for they have no power to move the hearts of men."

– Johann Wolfgang von Goethe

D tells you to **Dream Big, Dream Bigger,** and **Dream the Biggest Dream of All**. Never give up on your dreams. As children, we dream all of the time, and then life somehow manages to squash those dreams. Don't let life kill your dreams! Ask yourself, "Once I reach my goal weight, what one new thing will I do that I have never done before?" Now ask yourself, "Why wait? Why not do it now?!"

Maintain a dogged determination to fulfill your dreams by keeping the desire burning. Desire comes from setting *big* dreams, because small dreams do not have the power to move your heart. Devote yourself to the fulfillment of those dreams. They are your dreams, after all, and they will never be realized unless you strive to fulfill them. Don't die with your dreams unrealized. Today, make a plan to accomplish one of your childhood dreams.

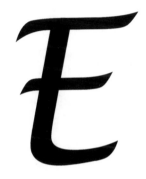

ELIMINATE CRITICISM, EMBRACE EMPATHY

"Consciously choose to smile, whenever it crosses your mind not to do so."

– Dr. Duc Vuong

E tells you to **Eliminate All Criticism**. To find compassion, you must eliminate all criticism. And the first form of criticism you need to eliminate is self-judgment. Stop judging yourself for the decision to have surgery or for putting yourself in the situation to even need surgery in the first place. Stop criticizing yourself because of the emotions you feel following your weight loss surgery. You're not weak or selfish, so don't criticize yourself. Let your long-suppressed buried emotions erupt if you have to; it's okay. Then look in the mirror and say, "I forgive you."

E also tells you to **Embrace Empathy**. Next, stop criticizing others. Understanding *your emotions* gives you empathy for others; forgiving *yourself* makes it easier to forgive others. Empathy allows you to relate to others in meaningful and sincere ways; it's the emotion we often fail to develop but the one that plays a major role in our success. In order to have empathy, you must purge all forms of criticism. Criticism is the cause of all unhappiness, so eliminate it. I will say that again: criticism is the cause of all unhappiness.

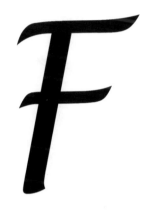

FORGIVENESS

"Forgiveness is the fragrance the violet sheds on the heel that has crushed it."

– Mark Twain

F is for **Forgiveness**. Nelson Mandela said, "Having resentment is like drinking poison and expecting your enemy to die." The only way to enlightenment is to forgive anything and everything that has happened to you in the past, however difficult this may be, for you can *never* have a better past. You must forgive the people and those events that you blame for your obesity.

"But how can I forgive when the pain is so much?" you ask. If you constantly think thoughts of forgiveness towards the one who has hurt you, then you will eventually feel forgiveness in your heart. Forgiveness must come from the heart, not the mind. After forgiving them, you must then send to them all of the things you wish for yourself, like love, peace, and prosperity.

Do not say "I will forgive, but I will never forget", because that is just another way of saying "I will not forgive." While it is impossible for you to have a better past, you can still control your future, so create a better future by forgiving the past.

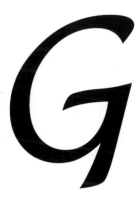

GIVING

"I have found that among its other benefits, giving liberates the soul of the giver."

– Maya Angelou

G takes you from *forgiving* to **Giving**. Many weight loss books will teach you to set goals and go for them. As a big believer in setting goals, I have set and achieved many big goals in my life. But in this book, I think it is more important that G stands for Giving rather than Goals. Oftentimes, obesity forces you to get others to do things for you that you can't or won't do for yourself. Consciously or unconsciously, you are a taker rather than a giver. To change the quality of your life, you must *give*, and define yourself as a *giving person*. If someone took advantage of your giving nature in the past, it reflects badly on them...not you; so don't let past betrayals be a reason for you to not be a giving person.

Obesity takes from you too. It robs you of your energy, your health, your loves, your opportunities. But paradoxically the antidote is *giving*—for whatever you give, you shall receive ten-fold. You don't have to give material things—you may give love, kindness, a compliment, or just a smile.

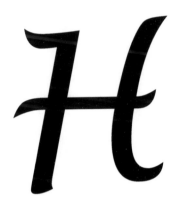

HUMILITY

"I claim to be a simple individual liable to err like any other fellow mortal. I own, however, that I have humility enough to confess my errors and to retrace my steps."

– Mahatma Gandhi

H is for Humility. Immediately after your weight loss surgery, you may be excited by your progress as the pounds just seem to melt away effortlessly. But you must remain humble. This is a personal journey, not a race against others. While some surgeons often brag about their patients' success as a percentage of weight lost, you and your surgeon must remember to remain humble and thankful for each ounce lost and every milestone reached. You will have periods where your weight loss will stall. Weight loss rarely proceeds in a straight line, so be humble as you face challenges. This is a life-long marathon, not a weekend sprint; it is measured in years, not months.

Humility should encompass every act or task that you endeavor. Humility is the backbone within which you eliminate criticism, and thereby can accomplish many great things. Practice being humble by giving thanks to the universe and those around you for the blessings in your life. Start each morning by saying, "Thank you, thank you."

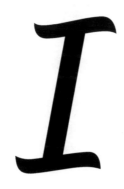

INNER PEACE

"The life of inner peace, being harmonious and without stress, is the easiest type of existence."

– Norman Vincent Peale

I is for Inner Peace because I believe that what every human being ultimately desires is inner peace. It's not easy to find, and people chase after it all the time. For example, they seek it in money, fame, or sexual conquests. But as Dr. Wayne Dyer says, the way to peace and happiness is in knowing that peace and happiness are the way. You must choose to be happy and choose to be at peace. Choose to be at peace with your current weight loss, your choice of weight loss surgeries, and your choice of surgeon.

You control your emotions. No one can make you feel any particular way. So don't think "He makes me so angry," or "She really knows how to push my buttons." Such thoughts rob you of your power. Control over your emotions is very powerful, so do not give away that power to anyone else. Choose to be at peace today—because yesterday has passed, tomorrow is uncertain, and all you really have is today. Have inner peace today.

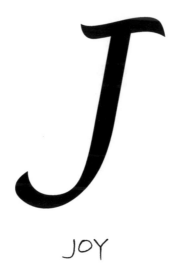

JOY

"Your success and happiness lies in you. Resolve to keep happy, and your joy and you shall form an invincible host against difficulties."

– Helen Keller

J stands for Joy. You have to find joy in the activities that your new healthier self requires. Sticking to any meaningful changes long-term will be difficult for you if you think that making healthier choices is a burden rather than a joy. If you think losing weight is a struggle, then losing weight will always be a struggle. If you don't celebrate your new body, then it won't be long before your old body returns. You will reap the rewards of your hard work if you do everything with a sense of joy. So discover one new activity today that you enjoy doing.

What is the difference between Joy and Happiness? The famous Buddhist monk, Thich Nhat Hanh, explains the difference like this: Imagine a man who is lost in the desert. Suddenly, he looks up and sees an oasis. His heart is filled with joy, even though he knows he must walk for another 15 minutes. Once he reaches the oasis and is able to drink and quench his thirst, he is happy. And therein lays the difference between joy and happiness. With joy, there is excitement. With happiness, there is peace.

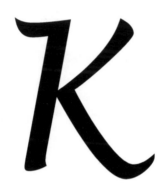

KNOWLEDGE

"Ignorance is the curse of God; knowledge is the wing
wherewith we fly to heaven."

– William Shakespeare

K is for **Knowledge**. Unlike the old saying, what you don't know *will* hurt you. You've got to acquire new knowledge. I don't give you much chance for success after surgery if you rely on the same old information. If you continue to think that beef jerky is a good snack, then I foresee weight struggles in your future. If you keep hoping that "low fat" or "fat-free" will make you healthy, I only see more disappointments headed your way. You have to read new and better books, watch better TV programs, hang out with better people who will inspire you. You have to take the classes, learn new skills, and challenge yourself to be better.

Patients often forget that you must exercise your brain in order to build it, just as you exercise your body. And you do this by giving your brain great books to read. Reading is like extreme CrossFit Cardio for your brain. You wouldn't feed your new body junk food, so don't feed your brain trashy books such as romance and Harlequin novels. Instead, choose books on gardening, cooking, self-improvement, financial literacy, success, and spirituality.

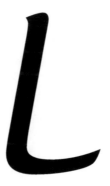

LOVE

"I have found the paradox, that if you love until it hurts, there can be no more hurt, only more love."

– Mother Teresa

L is for **Love**. Many patients sigh at the thought of having to give up their "favorite foods." Where have your old favorites gotten you? To weight loss surgery, that's where. Why would you waste another second pining over something that has kept you from the life you deserve? You need to find new favorites that you love and that love you back. You have to love your new body, your new self, your new soul because love is the basis of everything; the ultimate way. It is our ultimate mission in life to become beings of pure love, leading to inner peace. But this can only happen if we believe that we live in a *loving* world.

Love is the ultimate panacea and pacifier. It takes two people to fight, and you cannot fight with someone who no longer wishes to fight with you. So rather than fighting with the other person, send them love instead. You cannot be in a relationship with someone who no longer wants to be in a relationship with you. And this is true too for the "new you" and the "old you". Send the *old you* love, and release her to go along on her own merry way. Say, "I release the old me."

If you currently do not feel love in your life then you can change this by laughing. Laughter is the best medicine; it lifts your spirits and attracts love into your life. By being around those who make you laugh, you will increase the laughter in your world and you will find love. You will become love. Find a reason to laugh today.

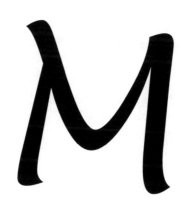

MINDFULNESS

"Don't be mind-less.   Be mind-full."

– Dr. Duc Vuong

M means **Mindfulness**. Life is too short to live it mindlessly; so become mind-full rather than mind-less. People often think that weight loss necessarily means changing your lifestyle. "Change your lifestyle" is said so often that it really has become an empty phrase these days. I really dislike it, so instead I say, "You have to change your *mind-style*."

Change. Your. Mind. Style.

Your new life starts with being mindful: mindful of your body and what you put in it; mindful of your thoughts and actions; and mindful of your place in this world. Think about the thoughts that you are having—are they positive or are they negative? Enhance your mindfulness today through the practice of mindful meditation. You can mindfully meditate during any activity, like walking, gardening, running, eating, or brushing your teeth by just being *in* the moment.

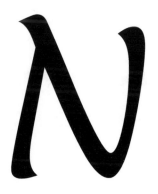

NOW

"People don't realize that now is all there ever is;
there is no past or future except as memory or
anticipation in your mind."

– Eckhart Tolle

N is for **Now** because you can only live in the Now. We all have moments of dwelling in the past or hoping for the future, but in actuality the Past and Future do not exist, except as a useful form of social convention. Truth is only the Present exists. The Past does not exist because everything that happened to you in the Past actually occurred in the Present. And everything that is going to happen to you in the Future, when it happens, will again only occur in the Present.

If you live in the Past, you live with regret and the risk of depression—like maybe you wonder how your husband could still be in love with someone who has become so obese. But dwelling in the Past does not improve your Future (because you can never have a better Past); it only robs you of your Today. If you live in the Future, you live with fear and doubt and anxiety about what the Future will hold—like possibly having excess skin after the surgery or regaining the weight. The only time you can control is *now*, so worry about controlling the future when it becomes the Now... as surely it will.

All we ever have is *Now*; so *live now*. Stop and focus only on what you are doing *Now*.

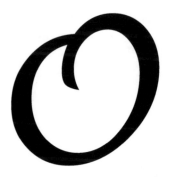

OPTIMISM

"Optimism is the faith that leads to achievement."

– Helen Keller

O is for **Optimism**. William James said that pessimism leads to weakness and optimism leads to power, so ask yourself, "Do I want to be weak or powerful? Doubtful or bold? Insecure or confident?" Obesity is pessimism incarnate, and one can quickly become a very pessimistic person when, after a night of restless sleep, waking each morning to the feeling of aching joints and the sight of a handful of pills. Rather than focusing on pessimistic predictions such as "I can't fit into that booth" or "I can't walk that far without a chair," try to look optimistically at your half-full glass: "I'm on my way. I'm making progress" or "I tried something new today." Opportunities for optimism abound, just waiting for you to reach out and seize them. Seize one today. Make a bold choice today. Think that your life is changing for the better.

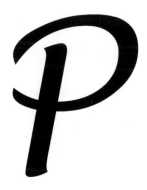

PERSEVERANCE

"Perseverance is not a long race; it is many short races one after the other."

– Walter Elliot

P is for **Perseverance.** Perseverance is often what distinguishes those who are successful from those who are not, not just with weight loss but with life in general. Picture the waves crashing against the rocks. The rocks are very hard, and the water is very weak, but the water is very persistent, and over the course of many centuries, the water will eventually win. Persevere through the last push-up, the last mile of the marathon, the long summer drought, the dark, cold, winter's night. Yes, you have to persevere, but you have to persevere towards your goals only in the present. The waves never stop and say, "Well, I persevered yesterday, so today I will take a break."

While perseverance implies a future payoff from your present pain, you cannot persevere in the future or the past. Rather than reliving past events as you drift off to sleep (...*should-have, could-have, would-have*...) realize that the past has already passed. Learn from your mistakes, but let go of past events and *persevere only in the present*. As you go through your day, do not think about the past or the future. Focus instead only on persevering in the present.

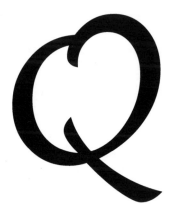

QUALITY, NOT QUANTITY

"The quality, not the longevity, of one's life is what is important."

– Martin Luther King, Jr.

Q is all about **Quality, not Quantity**. Obesity teaches us to value quantity over quality: the $1 menu over the carefully crafted cuisine; cheap cuts of meat instead of humanely and locally sourced; the heaping Friday Seafood Platter instead of the fresh catch of the day. I ask you to reverse this by starting to value quality over quantity. Buy only the best foods, settle for only the best organic produce, and go to only the nicest restaurants. Buy nicer clothes that fit well and will last longer; they will help you to feel better about yourself. Insist on interacting with only the best people, and value nourishing relationships above caustic ones. Remember, you become the average of your five closest relationships. So if your closest relationships are obese, you will most likely struggle with your weight. If they are living paycheck to paycheck, then you too are most likely struggling with your bills. If they have been divorced or have relationship issues, then most likely you have gone or will go through your own relationship heartaches.

Choose quality every time—in material possessions, relationships, and experiences—because ultimately you will get what you pay for. And know that you are worth the higher price.

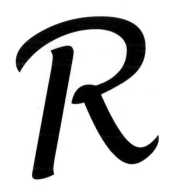

REASONING

"Most of our so-called reasoning consists in finding arguments for going on believing as we already do."

– James Robinson

R is for **Reasoning**, which is used in a bad sense here. Don't let your reasoning get the best of you. It is a bad habit, better described as bargaining. Some people call it *rationalizing*. It goes like this, "Well since I had a diet soda with lunch, I can have a cookie." Or "My blood sugar is too low, so I better have some chocolate milk." You have to be more resourceful than that. You have to plan for your success. Plan your work, work your plan, as the old saying goes.

Reasoning in this sense is toxic because it lulls you into a false sense of comfort. It encourages you to become complacent for the moment. "This one time won't hurt." "It's only half a slice..." "I'll go to the gym tomorrow." Then the one moment becomes *moments*, and before you know it a week has passed, then a month, then a season. And now your initial *comfort* has turned into *discomfort*. Discard those thoughts and behaviors that keep you tethered down, like your old habit of reasoning. Replace a reasoning thought today with one that is positive, like *Resourcefulness*.

S

SPIRITUALITY

"Know that you are a divine spiritual creature having a human experience, not a human who occasionally has a spiritual experience."

– Pierre Teilhard de Chardin

S is for **Spirituality**. After weight loss surgery, most patients treat the body like a temple by not littering it with junk food. However—you must not only develop your physical strength, but also your spiritual strength. Your new physical strength is your healthy body. Your new spiritual strength is your emotional fortitude. Spirituality means different things to different people. Find what it means for you. Do not judge what it might mean for others.

As far as we can tell, you are the most highly evolved creature in the universe. Your God, Spirit, Life Force, Energy—or whatever you choose to call it—did not put you here so that you could live a small and unfulfilled life. With your new found strength and courage, be spontaneous. Go do something you've never done before. Be bold. Make big choices. Be surprising. Wear the bathing suit. Go on an unplanned trip. Speak up in the meeting. Ask him on a date. You only have this life to live. Do not live it small. Know that you are a divine creature of God. Know that you are powerful beyond measure. Resolve to no longer live small. This confidence to live boldly is the true purpose of Spirituality.

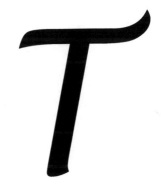

THOUGHT

"The ancestor of every action is a thought."

– Ralph Waldo Emerson

T stands for **Thought**. Everything begins with thought, and your thoughts are what ultimately determine your success or failure because it is through your thoughts that you create your reality. The small stories that we tell ourselves everyday— "I'm not pretty enough", "I'm not good at math", "I'm scared of heights", or "I can't cook or garden"—are all thoughts, and they are all lies. You can just as easily think the opposite: "I *am* beautiful", "I *am* strong", and "I *am* good at cooking." For example, thinking that you are good at cooking will make you more likely to watch a cooking show, or buy a cookbook, or try a new recipe. Thinking that you are smart might be the extra push you need to enroll back in college and finish your degree. Trusting in your ability to learn new skills will help you to redefine yourself as a new person. Instead of thinking that gardening is difficult, think to yourself "My thumb is getting greener." Then go out and learn the new skills that will actually make you a better gardener.

Every time you have a thought, ask yourself "Is this thought helping me or hurting me?" If it is hurting you, then you must get rid of it and replace it with a helpful thought. Do not try to justify negative thoughts with what I call *Yeah-but's*—"Yeah, but keeping it up will be hard", "Yeah, but my family will not like the new, healthy food choices", or "Yeah, but you don't know how bad I've had it." If a thought is not helping you, let it go, and then replace it with a positive one that will help you.

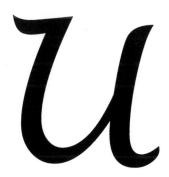

THE UNIFIED FIELD

"You and I are essentially infinite choice-makers. In every moment of our existence, we are in that field of all possibilities where we have access to an infinity of choices."

– Deepak Chopra

U means the **Unified Field**. We all come from the same stuff. Einstein's famous equation $E=MC^2$ tells us that mass and energy are equivalent; therefore we are all forms of energy. And since energy can never be created nor destroyed, our energy is indistinguishable from the energy in the wider universe—the energy that came into being at the time of the Big Bang or Creation. Our energy is the same energy that created the heavens and the stars. We all started as stardust, and we will all return to stardust.

Because everything that has ever existed or will ever exist was created during this initial event, anything you want, need or desire already exists in the energy field of possibilities, called the Unified Field. When a new skyscraper is built, many people mistakenly think that it "sprang up overnight" from nowhere, without realizing that all of the steel and concrete, all of the stuff that that skyscraper is made of was actually already here, just in a different form. Everything you've ever wanted is here for the taking, and you only have to ask.

As you are losing weight (mass), you are releasing energy back into the Unified Field, which is why you might feel tired right after your weight loss surgery. This energy gap must be rebalanced according to the laws of nature, and this rebalancing might take various forms: the pleasure of eating fresh fruits and vegetables, the excitement of a new promotion, or the passion of a new relationship. (Pleasure, excitement, and passion are all forms of energy.) You must be receptive to these changes, otherwise the excess energy will be converted right back into mass (your weight).

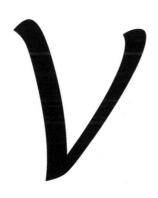

VECTOR

"Your time is limited, so don't waste it living someone else's life. Don't be trapped by dogma—which is living with the results of other people's thinking. Don't let the noise of others' opinions drown out your own inner voice. And most important, have the courage to follow your heart and intuition."

– Steve Jobs

V is for **Vector**, defined as a quantity moving in a direction; and in this case it is force. You must be that vector, that force going in a certain direction. Stay in motion always, because everything that is not actively growing or changing is dying or decaying. An acorn lying on the ground has the potential to become a giant oak tree, but it will die if it is unable to send out a tap root in the right direction. Even though it might look viable on the outside, an inactive acorn is actually a decaying acorn, just as your inactive soul is a decaying soul.

Use your voice as a vector to signal your departure from your old life (as a decaying acorn) towards your new life as a mighty oak. Don't speak with your old voice. Don't use your old words. Find new words. Find a new voice. Choose a new direction, and stay on that vector. Change and grow, or you will surely decay and die.

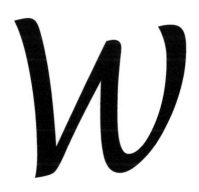

WHY'S

"He who has a why to live can bear almost any how."

– Friedrich Nietzsche

W is all about your **Why's**. Find your *Why's* because they will keep you going during tough times. *Why* did you have weight loss surgery? *Why* must you find new food favorites? *Why* are you rearranging your life? *Why* should you question every relationship in your life, including the relationship you have with yourself? Find your *Why's* and hold onto them. They are your compass, your purpose, your beacon in the night. Remember, it's not what you are eating…it's what's eating you, so figure out your *Why's*.

As new things come into your life, you will need new *Why's*, so regard these new events in a state of awe and wonderment. Do not question them or second guess them. Appreciate the new *Why's* that the Unified Field is bringing to you.

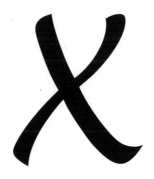

X-MEN®

"My weaknesses have always been food and men - in that order."

– Dolly Parton

X stands for **X-Men**®. Obesity sometimes makes us feel like mutants. But we all have a superhero within us, so find your hidden superhero. Unlock that superhero, for it is your true self. Like superheroes, we all have a special talent. Trust in that special talent. Tap into your talent by changing your thoughts. Think, "Who am I? Where did I come from? What am I meant to do?" The best superheroes struggle with these questions.

And all superheroes have a particular weakness—like Superman's susceptibility to Kryptonite. You must discover your weaknesses, and avoid them. I'm not talking about simple surface dieting weaknesses like "carbs" or "sweets" or "stress". I suggest you dig deeper for your weaknesses by asking yourself questions like "Why am I scared to express myself?" or "Why do I respond this way when that happens?" or "What could I accomplish if I really focused all of my energy on my goal?"

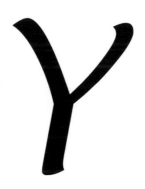

YOU

"Go confidently in the direction of your dreams. Live the life you have imagined."

– Henry David Thoreau

Y tells you to focus on **You**. You cannot serve others or take care of them, if you do not first take care of *you*. But this is not what society leads us to believe. We are all encouraged to put others before ourselves, but this doesn't really get us very far, does it? It is better to live as a shining example rather than die as a martyr who will quickly be forgotten. Many patients blame their obesity on the fact that they are "always doing for others before themselves." But how true is this really, since we cannot do much for others if we are sick ourselves?

While losing weight won't bring back your lost youth, you will discover a new "youthful" energy that must be enjoyed and appreciated; lest this energy be lost back to whence it came: the Unified Field. You must spend this new energy on *you*. The Unified Field is providing it to you so that you won't make the same mistakes that resulted in your obesity. Place yourself first, because *you* is all you've got. Do something nice for yourself today.

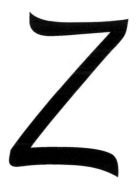

ZEN

"Meditation can help us embrace our worries, our fear, our anger; and that is very healing. We let our own natural capacity of healing do the work."

– Thich Nhat Hanh

Z is for **Zen**. Come to a place of peace, of Zen, through meditation. Find a new form of energy by meditating for 20 minutes twice a day, and these will be the best 20 minutes of your day. You will find yourself more refreshed, calmer, and ready to take on the day. But don't confuse meditation with prayer (which has a different purpose). Prayer is private communion with your God, whereas meditation is about trying to quiet your mind in order to tap into the realm of all possibilities: the Unified Field.

Find a form of meditation that works for you. Mindful meditation is a simple form that can be practiced anywhere. To begin, first set the timer on your phone for 10 minutes; then sit in quiet contemplation of your breath until the alarm sounds. When a stray thought enters your mind, just release it, and turn your attention back to your breath. Practice this until you can sit uninterrupted for increasingly longer periods of time. Try to slip into the gap between your thoughts—this is where you will find the Unified Field, which is the realm of all possibilities.

THE LAST WORD...

You have now reached the end of this book of 26 valuable lessons for weight loss success. But we never stop learning, and there are many more lessons still to be learned if you decide to become a lifelong learner. And there are many more applications of these lessons beyond weight loss, so try applying them to other aspects of your life.

While each lesson is important, my personal favorite lesson is *S for Spirituality*. Here is a quote from Marianne Williamson, which I love and wish to share with you.

"Our deepest fear is not that we are inadequate. Our deepest fear is that we are powerful beyond measure. It is our light, not our darkness that most frightens us. We ask ourselves, 'Who am I to be brilliant, gorgeous, talented, fabulous?' Actually, who are you not to be? You are a child of God. Your playing small does not serve the world."

– Marianne Williamson

Because you came from a higher power—whether you call it God, Allah, Yahweh, or Spirit—and because this higher power cannot make mistakes, then know that you were born perfect. Know that you have the power to make your life exactly as you wish it to be. When you are this powerful, fear does not exist. If fear does not exist, then stress does not exist. And if stress does not exist, then you are at peace. With inner peace, you find happiness, and you have an abundance of love to share.

Remember that your ultimate destiny in life is to become a being of pure love.

Blessings to you.

Dr. V

"For your tomorrows to come true, you must focus on your todays."

--Dr. Duc Vuong

"No one lays the bricks for your yellow brick road, except for you."

--Dr. Duc Vuong

About The Author

Dr. Duc Vuong is a bariatric surgeon and director of Lovelace Bariatrics in Albuquerque, New Mexico. He is an expert in the psychological aspects of obesity and has developed an intensive perioperative educational program that prepares his patients for success after weight loss surgery. He personally leads weekly educational groups, because understanding the individual struggles of his patients is essential to devising their best surgical program.

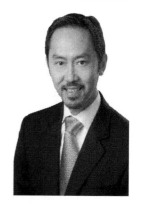

A popular speaker, Dr. Vuong has authored multiple patient-oriented weight loss surgery books and starred in the hit TLC show "900 Pound Man: Race Against Time."

Other Books by Dr. Duc Vuong:

Tighten Your Belt: *Overcome Obesity*

Ultimate Lap Band Success: *The Support Surgeon's Guide to Getting the Most from Your Gastric Band*

Ultimate Gastric Sleeve Success: *A Practical Patient Guide to Help Maximize your Weight Loss Results*

73931141R10035

Made in the USA
San Bernardino, CA
11 April 2018